I0435762

MINDFUL EATING

Have Your Cake and Eat It Too!

SHELLEY CHARLTON

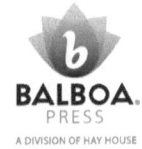

BALBOA
PRESS

A DIVISION OF HAY HOUSE

Copyright © 2017 Shelley Charlton.

All rights reserved. No part of this book may be used or reproduced by
any means, graphic, electronic, or mechanical, including photocopying,
recording, taping or by any information storage retrieval system
without the written permission of the author except in the case of
brief quotations embodied in critical articles and reviews.

Balboa Press books may be ordered through booksellers or by contacting:

Balboa Press
A Division of Hay House
1663 Liberty Drive
Bloomington, IN 47403
www.balboapress.com.au
1 (877) 407-4847

Because of the dynamic nature of the Internet, any web addresses or
links contained in this book may have changed since publication and
may no longer be valid. The views expressed in this work are solely those
of the author and do not necessarily reflect the views of the publisher,
and the publisher hereby disclaims any responsibility for them.

The author of this book does not dispense medical advice or prescribe the use
of any technique as a form of treatment for physical, emotional, or medical
problems without the advice of a physician, either directly or indirectly. The
intent of the author is only to offer information of a general nature to help you
in your quest for emotional and spiritual well-being. In the event you use any
of the information in this book for yourself, which is your constitutional right,
the author and the publisher assume no responsibility for your actions.

Any people depicted in stock imagery provided by Thinkstock are models,
and such images are being used for illustrative purposes only.
Certain stock imagery © Thinkstock.

Print information available on the last page.

ISBN: 978-1-5043-0904-2 (sc)
ISBN: 978-1-5043-0903-5 (e)

Balboa Press rev. date: 07/04/2017

Praise for *Mindful Eating: Have Your Cake and Eat It Too!*

"This book may be small, but it is very cute and full of love—just like the author."

Mike Dooley,
New York Times bestselling author

"A delicious read that will change your relationship with food. Your body will thank you!"

Andy Dooley,
Creator of Vibration Activation

"Shelley's philosophy has taken me almost a lifetime to discover for myself. The importance of enjoying our food—every mouthful—and to follow our instincts on what to eat make perfect sense. Oh, had I met her and read her book sooner. And I assure you, your weight stabilises, figure improves, and life holds so much more joy."

Carroll du Chateau,
Journalist and Restaurant Reviewer

"Shelley speaks from the heart in a fresh and honest way. Her real-world approach to mindful eating techniques is funny, real, and insightful. I do believe in the power of mindfulness and am excited about where nutritional genomics will lead us to better eating habits in the future."

Dr Kathleen,
IMD, Specialist in Integrative Medicine

"Sound advice for a healthier way to eat in a world where multitasking has become second nature to meet the demands of our busy lives."

Susan Bedford,
Artist and Intermediate/Advanced Mindful Eater

"Shelley writes with openness and honesty about a highly important topic that reminds us that how we choose to eat is almost as important as what we eat."

Jaqui Finlayson,
Nutritionist, Naturopath,
and Medical Herbalist

"Great food for thought! An insightful read by a genuine person."

Matthew Cattin,
Journalist

INTRODUCTION

Mindful Eating: Have Your Cake and Eat It Too! doesn't ask you to change what you're eating and drinking but to take a closer look at how and why you're eating and drinking. Besides, the new science is all about nutrigenomics, which investigates the foods that are best for you according to your genes. I'm sure you'll hear more and more about it in the years to come.

The game changer for me was a single line from Nadine Stair's poem, "If I Had My Life to Live Over Again," written when she was 85 years old. That line was, "I would eat more ice cream and less beans." I've been obsessed with diet and exercise all my life. There have been a few occasions when I completely let myself go due to traumatic events. Fortunately, I returned to health and fitness using the knowledge I had gained over the years. I have to admit this took extreme discipline and sacrifice. I figured there must be a better way.

In my twenties, I kept my weight under control with many hours in the gym or running for miles each week. In my thirties, I fell in love with yoga but found I had to cut down on the excessive amount of alcohol and ice cream I used to get away with. Now in my forties, I have finally learned to maintain a figure I am happy with by eating mindfully. At 45, I was mindful that I had no money in the bank. At 46, I was mindful that I was appearing on stage completely naked in *Calendar Girls*. And now, at 47, I am mindful that I am writing *Mindful Eating: Have Your Cake and Eat It Too!*

Joking aside, it has been so effective having my reason at the front of my mind before deciding whether to partake in treats. For example, I would stop and ask myself, "Do I really want to be spending money on extras when I'm already in debt?" "Do I really want the biscuits during rehearsals, or am I eating them just because they are there?" For me, mindful eating is all

about eating what you love and loving what you eat …
but only when you want to. I had a terrible habit of
eating for the sake of it until I learned the better way.
In this book, I've put together some of my thoughts,
observations, and results from experimenting in hope
you can learn to eat mindfully too.

BEGINNERS

This advice is backed up by science.

The greatest change you can make is to eat when you are relaxed. Our bodies are controlled by the autonomic nervous system, which is either in sympathetic mode (fight or flight) or parasympathetic mode (rest and digest). Basically, we're not meant to eat when we're stressed. When I say stressed, I don't mean on the verge of a nervous breakdown. I'm afraid we've all become used to the everyday stress that is, unfortunately, a way of life for most people. I would love to magically take away all your unnecessary stress, but for now, I suggest taking a few deep breaths just before you eat. Might seem a little weird to start with, but it's definitely worth a try.

Not too long ago, I spent a week with a colleague who checked her emails as she ate lunch each day.

The funny thing was, she had recently attended a mindfulness course. Priceless! As a kid, I always read whilst eating, even if it was the side of the cereal packet. I know it's usually a deeply ingrained habit, but if you could just concentrate on what you're eating and nothing else, I'm sure you'd soon notice an improvement in your digestion. There are some people I would not even dream of asking to get off the couch, sit at a table, and turn off the TV. Baby steps. However, why not pause the programme or turn the sound down to start with? When we're distracted whilst eating, we're hardly registering the food and are unlikely to feel satisfied.

For those who have moved away from the couch, how about setting up a nice area outside to enjoy meals? Granted, this may not always be suitable with weather conditions, but when it is, you'll find it's certainly worth the effort. If I can't be outside, I usually try to find a spot where I can gaze out the window. Nowadays, many people are eating at their desks, so at least select a scenic screen saver. Anything that makes you smile will work wonders.

To summarise:

1. Take a few deep breaths before eating.
2. Concentrate on nothing else but eating.
3. Eat in nature, or create a pleasant view.

INTERMEDIATE

This advice might seem a little woo-woo for some.

Once you've started to make a change using the previous suggestions, you're ready for these. They are evidence based but not necessarily widely known. A kale smoothie each morning may not be good for everybody. I definitely know it isn't for me. Once you take away the distractions, you can begin to listen to your body. When you start paying attention to your body, you'll eventually just know when something is or isn't right for you. I wasted a lot of time on tofu and cottage cheese. Never again.

To begin with, just notice how you feel after eating certain foods. If you feel congested, bloated, or have a runny nose, I'm guessing you could probably do without them, unless, of course, you absolutely love them and are happy to endure the after-effects.

Then go right ahead. I absolutely love bread. However, I get terrible wind after eating it! Doesn't mean I've given it up forever. Now I just pick when to have it, preferably when I don't have to teach a yoga class in the following 24 hours.

Before you eat something, ask yourself how you feel. Are you bored, angry, or sad? Then ask yourself the crucial question, "Will this food change the situation?" Highly unlikely. Is there something more productive you could do to improve how you feel? I used to rip open a big "party mix" bag of sweets as quickly as I could because I knew if I stopped to think about what I was doing, I'd realise I was just eating because I wasn't feeling too great. So take the time to check in with yourself. Try to fill your life with what's really missing instead of trying to fill your belly!

How often have you eaten something just because it was "on special" or free? I used to do my body a huge injustice by buying the cheapest option instead of having exactly what I wanted for a few dollars more. And don't get me started on the all-you-can-eat buffets! The whole point of eating mindfully is to eat what you love and love what you eat. If you buy the stale chocolate eclairs because they're half price, where's the love? Never eat for the sake of eating. Besides, eating cheap and nasty food will make your body crave the nutrients it requires, and you'll never feel satisfied. Just saying.

To summarise:

1. Listen to your body.
2. Check in with how you feel before you start eating.
3. Choose quality over quantity and bargains because you're worth it.

ADVANCED

This advice is admittedly "out-there."

This may be hard to believe, but your thoughts and feelings about the food you are eating affect the chemicals produced in your body and how the food is digested, used, and stored. I believe this explains why certain people live long and healthy lives despite eating what would normally be considered inadequate diets, whereas others who strive to eat as well as possible suffer from digestive problems or even worse.

For me, everything comes down to love or fear. Are you eating certain foods because you love and want them, or are you eating them because you're afraid of getting cancer or dying prematurely? Anita Moorjani explains this beautifully in her first book, *Dying to Be Me*. When I sit down to eat, I take a few breaths and think, *Thank you for this wonderful food, which serves* my *highest health and happiness*—even if it's the biggest bowl of boysenberry ripple ice cream you've ever seen!

If you can't get your head around the previous suggestion, maybe the thought of using energy works better for you. As a Reiki practioner, I have been taught to reiki my food and drink to increase its nutritional value, especially if a microwave has been used. This can be done by simply hovering your hands over your meal with the loving intention that the universal life force energy (prana/chi/ki/the field) will raise the vibration of what you're about to eat. I did say that this chapter was "out-there." However, what have you got to lose?

If you're still reading, there is a high probability you've seen the movie *What the Bleep Do We Know?* Maybe you remember the deaf actress who starts off not liking herself but gradually turns her life around with self-love. It is heavily based on quantum physics, and from what I can gather, our deep-rooted beliefs affect every single cell in our bodies as well as our genes. To learn more about epigenetics, Bruce Lipton's *A Biology of Belief* is a must-read. Also, check out this YouTube video, *Water, Consciousness & Intent: Dr Masaru Emoto* (https://youtu.be/tAvzsjcBtx8), which highlights Dr Emoto's work in the study of the relationship between water and words/intentions.

Most mornings I practise a short gratitude meditation before I get out of bed. I start off with, "Thank you for my beautiful toes, thank you for my beautiful feet," and so on, all the way through my body. All I know is that on those particular days, life is better. I feel more loving, more tolerant, and more compassionate towards myself and others. Sure, there are weeks when I feel more "squidgy" than others, but on the whole, I have learned to love my body just the way it is. And I sincerely hope you can learn to feel the same way!

To summarise:

1. Believe what you're eating is good for you.
2. Reiki your food.
3. Learn to love your body just the way it is.

CHALLENGE

For three days in a row, make notes on how and why you're eating. If you prefer, monitor your body's reaction to what you consume. The main objective is to pay attention to your body for at least 72 hours. If you give up after half a day, wait and start again another day. Give yourself this time to tune into you.

ACKNOWLEDGEMENTS

I would first like to say a huge thank you to my co-star in the stage play *Calendar Girls*. Greg and I have done a few shows together, and when he asked me one night during rehearsal what I was doing to lose weight, I replied, "It's the Mindfulness Diet … mindful that I'm broke!" And so, an idea was born.

Massive amounts of love and gratitude to the wonderful group I travelled with to Tahiti in March 2017. They were inspiring and supportive, and they provided crucial feedback.

A lot of what is stored in my subconscious is thanks to Jennifer Mclean's *Healing with the Masters* talk show and her extremely knowledgeable guests.

And finally, thank you for the Hay House World Summit! I have learned so much over the past few years and still manage to bewilder my friends with the latest discoveries.

NOTES

NOTES

NOTES

NOTES

NOTES

NOTES

NOTES

NOTES

NOTES

NOTES

NOTES

NOTES

NOTES

NOTES

NOTES

NOTES

NOTES

NOTES

NOTES

Author Bio

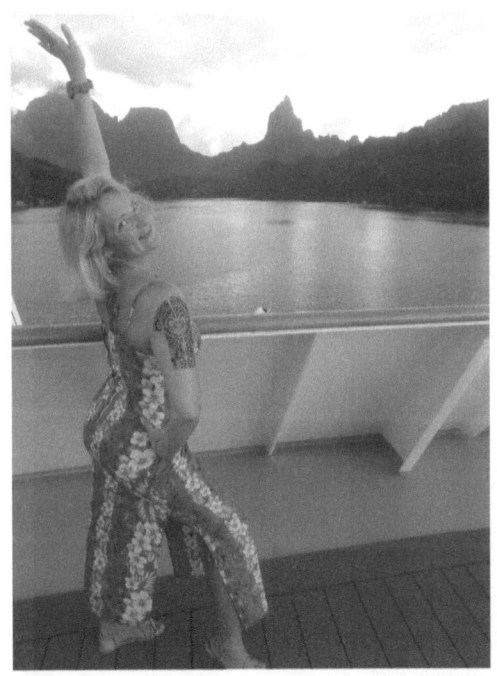

Shelley Charlton is an eternal student of Health, Wealth, and Happiness. After 17 years in the Air Force, she retired early to pursue her passions of acting and yoga. Shelley is currently living the dream on the Hibiscus Coast in New Zealand with her beloved cat, Puss.

www.ingramcontent.com/pod-product-compliance
Lightning Source LLC
Chambersburg PA
CBHW030544290526
45786CB00004B/1859